Essential Oils 40+:
The Top 40 Anti-aging Essential Oils To Feel And Look Perfect

Table of Contents

Introduction: A Great Looking Exterior

We would all like to look years younger, but for most of us, this usually seems like an impossible dream. But what if I was to tell you that all you need to keep your skin clear and without wrinkles can be found packed in a small little bottle of Essential Oil? This is no gimmick my friend, because essential oil is the extracted essence from healing herbal plants in its most potent form.

When these are used on the skin, they can have incredibly healing and rejuvenating effects. In reality the main cause of aging is a deficiency in the body. If we lack calcium, for example, as we get older this deficiency in calcium can cause our bone to become brittle until we are hunched over little old men and ladies from this very specific lack. The same can be said of our skin, often enough, cracked and aging skin is simply in need of vitamins being replenished.

So it is that by applying essential oils to our skins we are not adding anything that our bodies do not already need, we are simply replenishing what it has already lost. These oils are just a means of naturally altering the faltering chemistry of our exteriors! So in order to get your exterior self looking great, keep reading, and give essential oils a try.

Chapter 1: Anti-Aging Essential Oils that speed up Your Metabolism

Yes, one of the biggest bummers as we get older is a slowing metabolism. When you were 20 years old you could singlehandedly devour a whole pizza and not gain any weight but by the time you are 40 just eating one slice of pizza seems like enough to wreck your whole figure. There is just no way around it, our metabolism tends to slow down with age. But there are essential oils you can use with anti-aging properties that greatly mitigate these effects. Here are some of the best.

Prickly Pear Oil

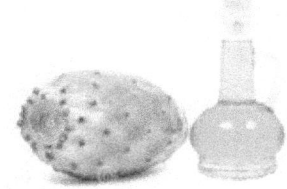

This essential oil is derived right from the seeds of the prickly pear cacti. In the process of extraction, this herb goes through an elaborate cleansing routine in wish the seeds are separated from the pulp and then washed very carefully. They then have all of this fantastic oil pressed right out of them. This oil can then be used to work wonders for the body's metabolism.

Just rub a small amount of this substance onto your skin and through absorption and good old fashioned aromatherapy your metabolism will almost instantaneously react. Prickly pear is not the first thing people might think of when it comes to reversing the effects of an aging metabolism but this anti aging essential oil can really do wonders.

Grapefruit Oil

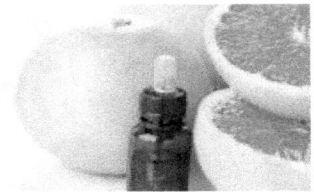

Most of you are probably more familiar with the grapefruit that we eat and drink. But let me tell you something, the oil that can be extracted from this edible herb, is even better than any tasty grapefruit cocktail. Grapefruit actually has at its disposal a very powerful fat busting agent that works upon the liver in order to burn up fat as soon as possible.

Regular use of this oil has also been shown to regulate blood sugar, and many other metabolic processes. So if you feel like age has caused your metabolism to slow down, just take a bit of this oil on your skin and utilize its fantastic anti aging properties. Grapefruit gives you the edge that you need, so go ahead and apply this wonderful anti aging essential oil to your metabolic needs and you will be ready to go.

Seaweed Oil

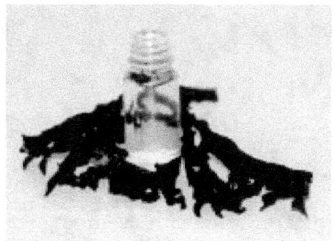

Yes, it may sound funny, but oil extracted even from seaweed can have some powerful effects on the human metabolism. This is a little known fact that the people of Japan have been privy to for quite some time. Seaweed oil is beneficial to our metabolism because of the heavy amount of iodine that it is composed of. This hearty helping of iodine has a great reaction upon our thyroid gland helping to directly boost our metabolism.

I couple of years ago I had an issue with my own thyroid gland, I was sure my doctor would give me all kinds of treatment, but instead he simply directed me the local health food store and told me to get some seaweed essential oil. After I spent the few dollars to get the small vial of essential oil I started using it on a regular basis and noticed a difference almost immediately. If you are having similar thyroid problems with your metabolism, I would recommend using this essential oil as soon as possible.

Gurmar Oil

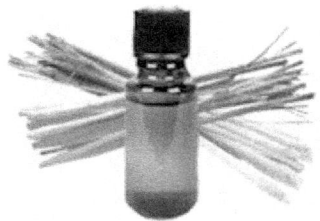

This essential oil has been used in India as a part of Ayurvedic medicine for thousands of years. It is the gymnemic acid inside of this oil that does so much to control appetite and kick start metabolism. If you have a problem with overdoing the sweets, and wrecking your blood sugar levels, Gumar oil can be a great metabolic aid to keep those cravings in check. I've known many people who were afraid of wrecking their diet and their metabolism from having a bad habit of eating too many sweets. All of them agree that after applying just a few drops of gumar essential oil, there sweet tooth problems are all taken care of.

Peppermint Oil

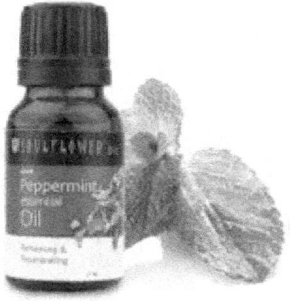

It is minty, and it is fresh, it coats candy canes every year at Christmas, and it also boosts metabolism! Common peppermint oil works well at cleansing the body of digestive ills such as bloating and upset stomach, while it simultaneously gives your overall metabolic process a tremendous boost. The anti aging metabolic properties of this essential oil will definitely make you feel a whole lot younger. The best way to use this peppermint essential oil is simply to smell it. It's so strong that I usually just take one small vial and put it underneath my nose and give it a good, strong whiff.

Hawthorn Oil

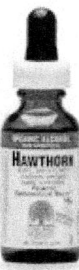

Oil extracted from the Hawthorne herb has been known to strengthen many metabolic processes of the body as we age. One of the great boons in this is the ability of this oil to strengthen the heart and general blood flow throughout the body. But as well as these vital functions, hawthorn oil can also boost the metabolism of those who apply it. Metabolism is like a tightly wound clock, you have to keep it perfect synchronization in order for it to work. Hawthorn oil works to keep your metabolism in sync.

Fennel Oil

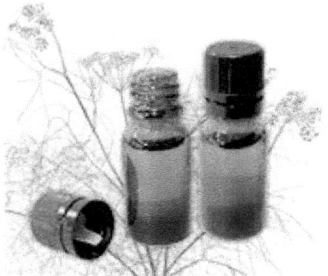

This essential oil is a powerful dietary aid, helping with all kinds of digestive and metabolic processes in the body. It has a strong licorice flavor and is able to be distributed through incense, provoking a strong aroma that opens up the airways and goes straight to the brain, instantly activating metabolic boosting health.

Chapter 2: Essential Oils for Wrinkles Stretch Marks and Cellulite

We all get wrinkles and creases on our skin. These form from simple repeated stress and wear and tear in our natural environment. So let's take some essential oils right back out of that natural environment and use them to supply our bodies with what they need. In this chapter let's take a look at some of the best essential oils to combat wrinkles and cellulite.

Geranium Oil

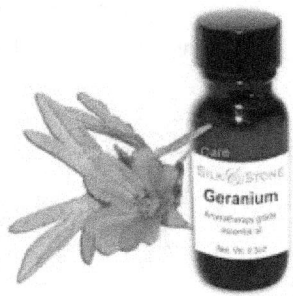

Extracted directly from the Geranium flower this oil is known for its ability to rejuvenate aches and pains, and curing constant fatigue syndromes that people suffer from. Geranium is known to greatly elevate the mood of those that use it. But as well as all of these features, when you apply geranium oil directly to the face it will work to smooth away wrinkles and lines as well.

So if you would like to streamline that face, you should definitely give geranium oil a try. By rubbing geranium essential oil directly into the skin, it will work to smooth away all of those cracks and fractures on your outer epidermal layers. Geranium essential oil is a fantastic anti aging agent that really works.

Aloe Vera Oil

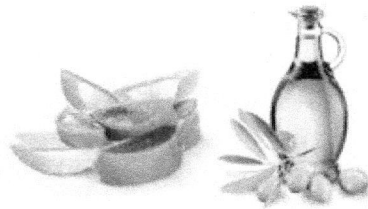

This healing oil is soothing to the skin on contact. Known for treating burns, whole burn wards at hospitals are constantly stocked with this stuff for its healing properties. But even if you are not a burn victim, the soothing oil from the Aloe Vera Plant can work wonders on your wrinkles as well.

Because in the end most wrinkling is essentially damaged skin anyway, all you have to do is put some of this oil on your skin and you will see the benefit almost immediately. This essential oil is fairly easy to come by too. You can by it readily made at most drug and health food stores, and you can also grow your own Aloe Vera plants yourself, harvesting the essential oil straight from the Aloe Vera leaves. It works great either way!

Sandalwood Oil

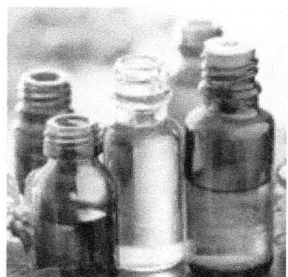

With a great woody aroma, sandalwood oil is often used as an active part of Ayurvedic medicine for quite some time. The oil is extracted directly from the sandalwood tree in places such as India, Australia, and Hawaii. This essential oil is known for its ability to fight the fog of aging, busting right through those wrinkles, and lines in no time! This is precisely why so many eastern religions have used sandalwood for their incense in their meditation, prayer; it gives them an ageless form of invigoration, coupled with a face lift!

If you ever wonder why the folks at the monastery look so young, it is no doubt due to the use of sandalwood oil! This essential oil has such powerful anti aging powers that it smooth's over even the most dry, cracked, and wrinkled skin! I especially use sandalwood oil in the winter months when the cold weather makes the skin on my hands cracked and dry. This essential oil is great for anyone who wants to keep their skin nice and smooth!

Rosewood Oil

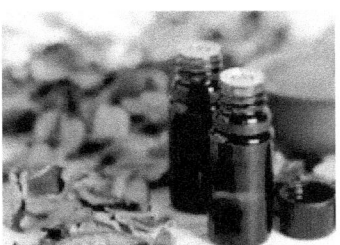

Extracted directly from the Aniba rosaeodora, a tree that is native to Peru, this essential oil is a great aid to eliminating stretch marks, wrinkles, and even cellulite. So if you feel like father time is starting to take a toll on your skin, then you should take some of this essential oil for some soothing restoration, right away! Rosewood oil really packs a punch and takes a bite out of the aging process. If your skin is starting to show wear and tear, or you have some pesky stretch marks that you would like to get rid of, just rub this essential oil directly into the skin and see these unsightly marks get rubbed right out of your life.

Avocado Oil

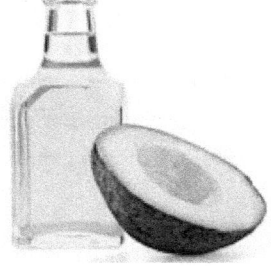

The avocado is actually known as a brain food and it is used as a great essential oil that enriches the skin. This oil happens to contain both folate and vitamin which are very important in the maintenance of your skin's dermatology. This is why so many have used a batch of avocados in their face treatments for so many years. A steady dose of this oil will do much to improve skin tightness and smoothness. Using avocado oil on the skin, has been a beauty secret for a long time, so you might as well add this essential oil to your anti aging arsenal.

Chapter 3: Anti Aging for Your Immune System

Unfortunately, for most of us our immune systems start to wind down as we get older. This means that for many the flu and cold season can really become quite a nightmare when you have an immune system that is faltering. But there is good news my friends, because there are some really wonderful essential oils that can boost that faltering immune system right back to its youthful integrity. Here are just a few of these anti aging immune boosting oils.

Echinacea Oil

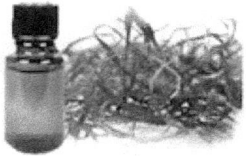

Working as a great anti-biotic and anti-viral agent, having some Echinacea oil works as a great boon when it comes to helping the immune system out against the threats that the environment throws at it. And so as we age, it would do you a whole lot of good to give your immune system the advantage that Echinacea oil can provide. Long used by native Americans for healing and enrichment of the immune system, Echinacea oil can make you strong enough to face just about anything that comes your way.

Astragalus Oil

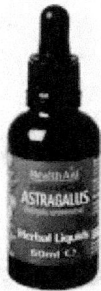

Dating back about thousands of years, this herb in its oil extracted form can work to boost the immune system. Just apply the oil directly to the skin and you can begin to immediately benefit from its potent power. This essential oil has been used by the Chinese for centuries, and has been consistently one of the best known ways of battling a troubled immune system. Use this essential oil today in order to find out how to start feeling a whole lot better tomorrow!

Saffron Oil

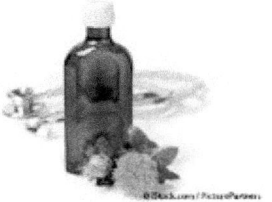

This essential oil helps to fight against depression as well as doing a lot to boost the immune system. The oil is taken directly from this herb's stem and applied directly to the skin. Saffron oil is a great anti aging agent for our immune system and should be used as much as needed. This essential oil is a potent yet non invasive treatment for whatever might be troubling you. Use some essential oil to bolster your immune defenses before it's too late.

Oregano Oil

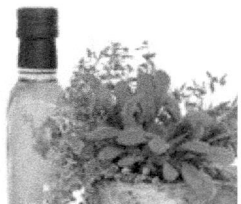

Oregano is loaded with free-radical fighting antioxidants. It is the free radicals floating around in our cells that cause much of the molecular breakdown associated with aging. And this couldn't be truer when it comes to the immune system as well. Oregano essential oil offers many great benefits and boosts to the immune system by bolstering its defense against dangerous bacteria, viruses and other microscopic organisms. Oregano is not just for your pasta sauce! It works well to boost your immune system too!

Ginger Oil

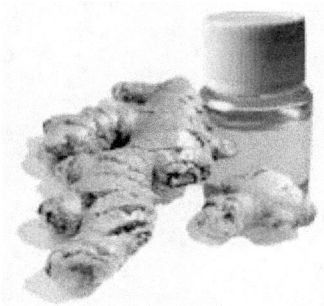

If you have joint trouble, ginger oil could do you a lot of good for your aching joints, this is due to the phytochemicals that are inside of the this essential oil which work as a great anti-inflammatory agent. These anti-inflammatory properties are good to bolster that faltering immune system as well. If you feel a little bit more prone to illness as you age, you should try to supplement your aging immune system with a ginger essential oil regimen today. Ginger oil is a healthy way to make sure that your immune system is working at its very best level.

Eucalyptus Oil

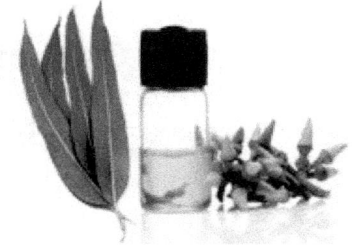

Just spread the aroma of this essential oil in the air and it will be enough to go right to the brain and activate cerebral activity. As soon as this soothing aroma is inhaled, you will find yourself refreshed and thinking much clearer. Eucalytus essential oil is one of the best ways to refresh your entire immune system all in one fresh eucalyptus breath!

Frankincense Oil

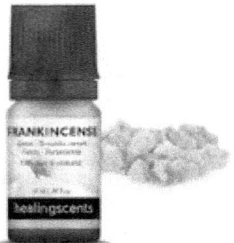

Now that we are close to the holiday season, you may remember the Christmas story of the three Kings of the East who bore the baby Jesus a gift of Frankincense and Myrrh. Well just like the original Christmas story depicts it, these two essential oils have been prized much more than their weight in gold for thousands of years.

Frankincense in particular works well to cleanse the whole body of outside pathogens and boost its immune defense. If you feel that the aging process has worn down your immune system, then by all means, you should give frankincense oil a try. If it was good for the three wise kings of Christmas then it can be good for you to!

Melaleuca Alternifolia

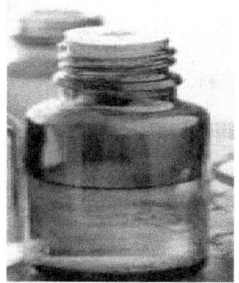

Just burn this powerful essential oil in an incense diffuser and you can feel the results as it enhances your body's immune system and its power of defecting illness. If you feel that as you grow older your immune system is failing, just give this oil a try! This essential oil works on a holistic level, taking care of the body's complete immune system health.

Chapter 4: Essential Oils For Young and Healthy Hair

We tend to place a lot of value on the health of our hair. There are expensive shampoos and treatments that are supposed to improve our hair follicles and scalp, but you can also get much the same (or better) results from a highly concentrated batch of essential oils. So here they are in no particular order, the best essential oils for young and healthy hair!

Lavender Essential Oil

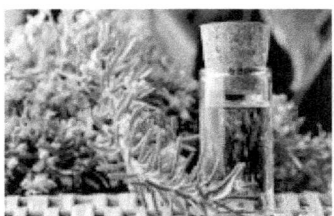

Extracted straight from the Lavender flower, this oil is soothing to the scalp and hair. When applied directly, this oil can actually help promote the circulation of blood in the scalp which in turn will help to improve growth, and serve as preventative maintenance against losing your hair. Lavender oil also serves to keep the roots of your hair moist and brings equilibrium to sebum production. This oil also works as a powerful antimicrobial agent, helping to eliminate dandruff and even acne from your scalp. With your sebum production enriched and balanced, lavender oil serves to make your entire head of hair young and healthy.

Rosemary Essential Oil

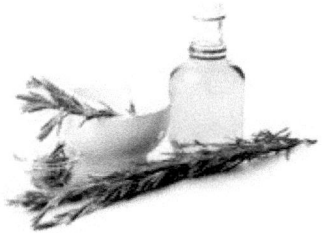

This woody scented essential oil is just loaded with antioxidants that do a great work of preventative maintenance when it comes to fighting the spread of gray hair. This oil when rubbed directly into the roots of your hair works to stimulate the hair follicles, reinvigorating them and bolstering them against losing their color. This oil also works to significantly clear up any clogging that might be happening in the pores of your scalp, preventing, dandruff, acne and other discomforts. This exfoliation will bring you healthy hair with a much younger sheen, just like you always wanted. So if your hair has been diminished by age, just use this essential oil to restore it to its youthful greatness.

Chamomile Essential Oil

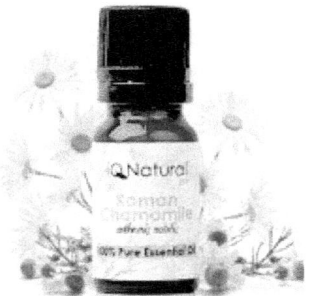

Chamomile essential oil has great anti-inflammation properties, and just by rubbing it directly into your hair you can get rid of dandruff, strengthen the hair follicles, and even enhance your hairs own natural coloring. Chamomile essential oil works to strengthen the hair keeping it from being damaged by external contaminates. Strengthening and nurturing it as you age. The anti aging properties of chamomile essential oil are absolutely phenomenal. Try this soothing and enriching anti aging essential oil and see the results for yourself!

Cedar Essential Oil

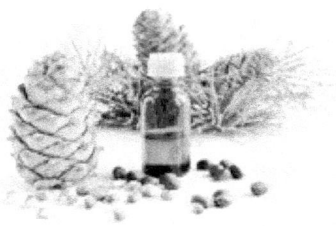

Cedar essential oil, especially extracted from the woody herb of the Cedrus Atlantica Tree, this essential oil works wonders against dandruff, and has even known to reverse the effects of thinning and balding hair. This essential oil helps to balance out the hairs own natural *sebum oil* allowing hair to dry out when it is too oily and to oil up when it is too dry. It also helps to promote the circulation of blood and the stimulation of hair follicles, enabling the vigorous growth of beautiful, and youthful full hair. You can simply add a few drops of this oil to your shampoo and massage it directly into the scalp as you wash your hair. You should see results almost immediately.

Clary Sage Essential Oil

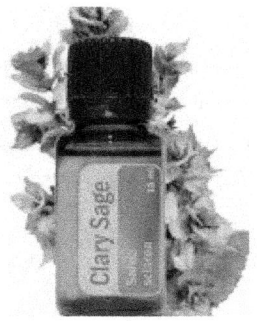

This essential oil has great value when it comes to its phyoestrogen content, a factor that can help promote hair growth in those who rub this oil into their scalp. This oil works well as a preventative measure against balding. It also works to help minimize dandruff and other excesses of an excessively oily scalp. If your hair is becoming particularly thin with age, this essential anti aging oil can really get your hair to thicken up. This essential oil will give your hair a silky and youthful sheen, just mix a few drops of this essential oil with your shampoo and apply it directly to the scalp.

Thyme Essential Oil

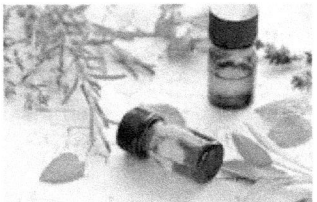

This spicy smelling oil can help to restore damaged hair, increase blood circulation, and generally enhance healthy hair growth. Thyme also has great antimicrobial properties that work as a direct anti aging agent against irritated and weathered scalps. Rubbing this essential oil directly into your scalp will deliver many important vitamins and nutrients that are crucial to hair development. These vitamins and nutrients are absorbed directly into the skin on contact. Thyme is also a cleansing agent and removes all dirt, dandruff, and excessive oil upon contact.

Lemon Essential Oil

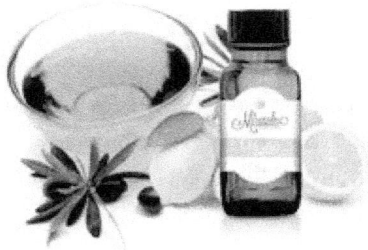

This essential oil works well for those of us that are plagued with an oily scalp as we get older. Lemon oil naturally works to dry out the scalp, preventing oily pimples from forming, and excessive dandruff. Lemon essential oil also naturally lighten hair if you would like to lighten up your hair color. Lemon oil calms and stimulates at the same tie while it puts the entire scalp into detox. All you have to do is add a few drops to your shampoo and you can see the results for yourself.

Patchouli Essential Oil

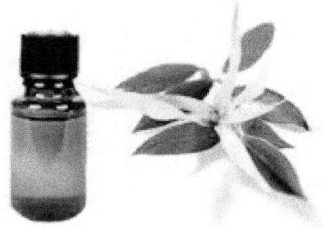

Alright, I know you guys have worn it at some point. There is an inner hippie in all of us that just loves the fragrance of this potent oil. But as well as providing us with some funky aroma's patchouli oil when applied directly to the scalp can also provide some great anti aging properties as well. This oil can help to treat a wide variety of age related ailments to the hair such as dry scalp, dandruff, dermatitis, and even eczema. If you are having any age related difficulty with your hair at all, this anti aging oil can get you right back on the right track once again.

Tea Tree Essential Oil

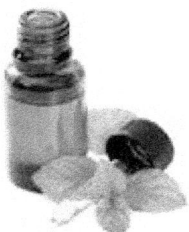

This oil can help alleviate almost any age related condition to the hair. It works wonders for dandruff and dry scalp. This oil when it is massaged directly into the roots of your hair works to completely unclog hair follicles and it even kills all bacteria as it cleanses. This simple essential oil has been proven and tested when it comes to creating healthy and youthful hair.

Vetiver Essential Oil

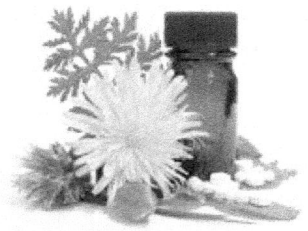

This oil has a great cooling effect as soon as it is put on the scalp, and promotes hair growth even as it relaxes hair right in the follicle. This is great when it comes to shielding your hair from premature aging from external environmental factors. Vetiver gives the hair a very special radiance and extra volume in order to combat the aging process.

Ylang Ylang Essential Oil

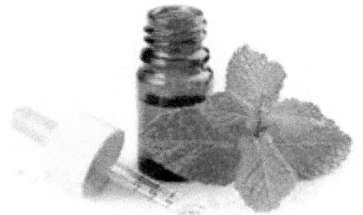

This essential oil helps to stimulate sebum production and eliminate dryness, allowing for much fuller and healthier hair. This oil also serves to bring equilibrium to hormone imbalances, allowing your hair to stay young and strong like it should be. This essential oil is all you really need in order to have healthy and well balanced hair.

Chapter 5 Anti Aging Essential Oils for Memory and Mental Clarity

It can be quite heartbreaking to see the ones that we love begin to struggle with memory loss and lack of focus in their lives. Yet, sometimes just the smell of a notable scent such as a certain brew of coffee or a sweet desert can trigger our memories. There are some fabulous essential oils that can boost your memory and focus. Let's go over them now.

Bergamot Essential Oil

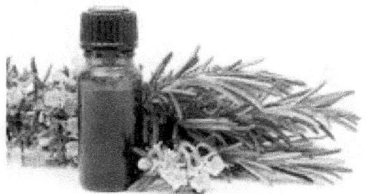

Bergamot has long been used to enhance mood, ad bring about mental clarity. Bergamot relieves anxiety and agitation and gives those who use it the ability to focus on their day. Just place a few drops of this essential oil into a incense burner and take a deep breath because with it, your mental clarity will return in no time. This essential oil can also do quite a bit when it comes to the age old problem of memory loss, so if you feel your memory start to slip, just take a few drops of this essential oil and you will be in some really great shape.

Coconut Essential Oil

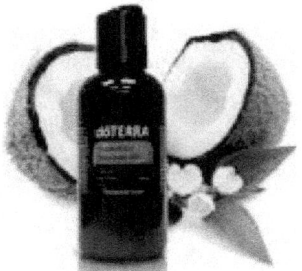

This essential oil ha been known to lift the fog of old age completely and bring about a restoration of memory for those who use it. Coconut oil has even been used to treat Alzheimer's and many other cognitive illnesses that are quite commonplace during the aging process. So if you are feeling a little bit less focused and your memory begins to slip, I would definitely give coconut oil a try. Coconut oil works to enrich your memory and to greatly enhance mental clarity and focus in those who use it.

Basil Essential Oil

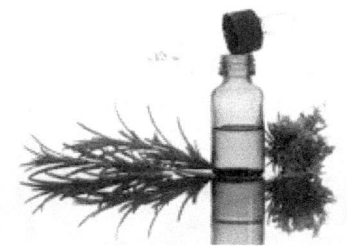

Just the aroma of basil essential oil has been known to work as an aid toward memory enhancement. Even many college students have vouched to the voracity of this oil and have used it right before exams in order to improve their recall before testing. Many claim that by just inhaling Basil before study sessions, or testing they have been able to greatly increase their retention of information. If you need help with your memory and focus, you should give basil a try. Basil is about as wholesome an as invigorating as it can be when it comes to helping memory and focus.

Cyprus Essential Oil

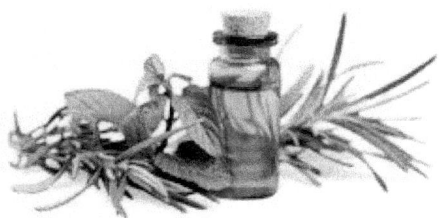

The evergreen scent of Cyprus is refreshing, and while it tends to trigger my memory of Christmas trees, this is not the only use for this oil. Cyprus oil when rubbed into the skin and inhaled can greatly increase concentration and focus. This essential oil is great for helping your memory and your ability to focus, if you think that age is causing either one of these cognitive abilities to decline then you should go ahead and give this Cyprus oil a shot.

Jasmine Essential Oil

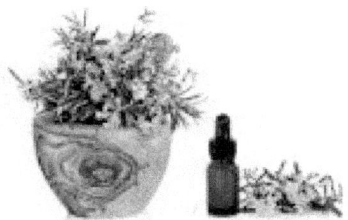

The smell of jasmine brings back pleasant memories for many, and this is especially the case when it comes to jasmine essential oil. Just breathe the oil and you will be inundated with a special aroma that will cast out all fatigue and bring a state of mental clarity back to those who use it. This essential oil can really do wonders for the mind, especially when it comes to memory support and cognitive function. Just apply a few drops of this oil and you will soon see some improvement in your condition.

Neroli Essential Oil

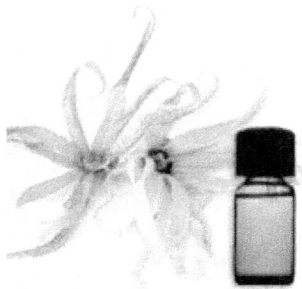

Neroli has an ability of decreasing the heart rate and bringing calm focus back into your life. If you feel a bit overwhelmed as you get older, use this anti aging treatment to bring clarity and focus back into your life. Just rub a few drops into your temples and you will soon have a restored memory, focus and clarity like never before. Neroli oil has been around a long time and will help you keep your memory going strong as long as you use it.

Rose Essential Oil

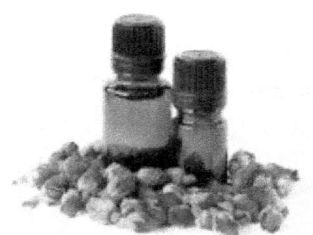

Rose oil helps to sooth the mind and bring back that clarity that you were missing. As you age you should boost your memory and focus with this great essential oil. It only takes a few drops of rose oil to see a difference, so if you would like to enhance your memory and other cognitive functions, use this essential oil as needed.

Grapefruit Essential Oil

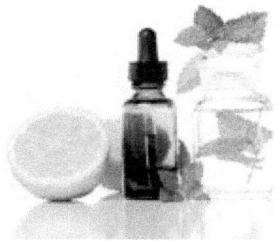

This essential oil gives you a great jumpstart to your memory and mental clarity. Enriching and vitalizing your brain cells and even the blood flow or your brain, greatly enhancing recall and focus. Something as sweet as grapefruit oil can really make a difference when it comes to memory and the aging process.

Coriander Essential Oil

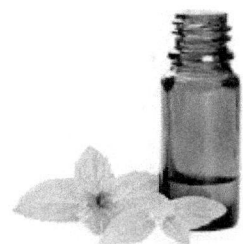

This essential oil can work as a great stimulating agent for your cognition even while it simultaneously calms the nerves. The blood circulation it promotes in the brain can help to improve memory and enhance focus. There is definitely a place for this oil when it comes to aging and wellness.

Conclusion: The Best Essential Oil Treatment

Aging really effects are lives in a variety of ways, but if you have the right resources at your disposal, you can work to greatly minimize these effects. We all age but we don't all age the same. And if you have the right combination of essential oils at work for you, you will be able to keep the bay the aging process at bay, because the best anti aging treatment is the best essential oil treatment.

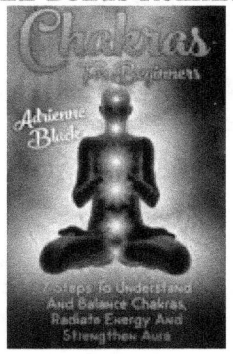

Simply Click the Button Below

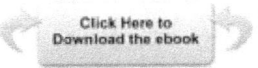

OR Go to This Page

http://lifehacksworld.com/free

BONUS #2: More Free & Discounted Books & Products

Do you want to receive more Free/Discounted Books or Products?

We have a mailing list where we send out our new Books or Products when they go free or with a discount on Amazon. Click on the link below to sign up for Free & Discount Book & Product Promotions.

=> Sign Up for Free & Discount Book & Product Promotions <=

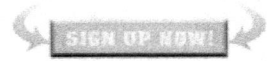

OR Go to this URL

http://zbit.ly/1WBb1Ek